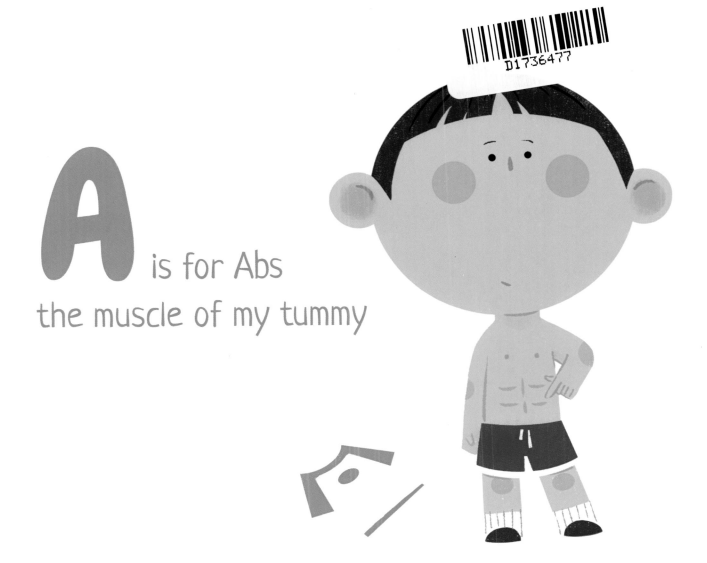

A is for Abs
the muscle of my tummy

B is for Burpees

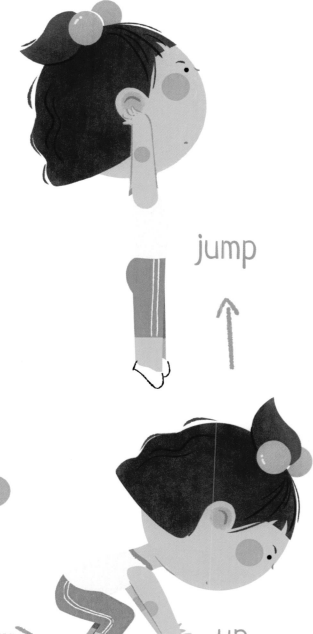

jump

↑

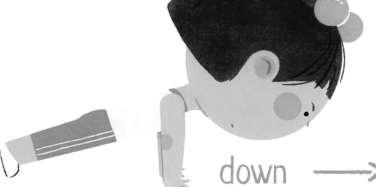

down →

up

C is for Cartwheel
round and round we go

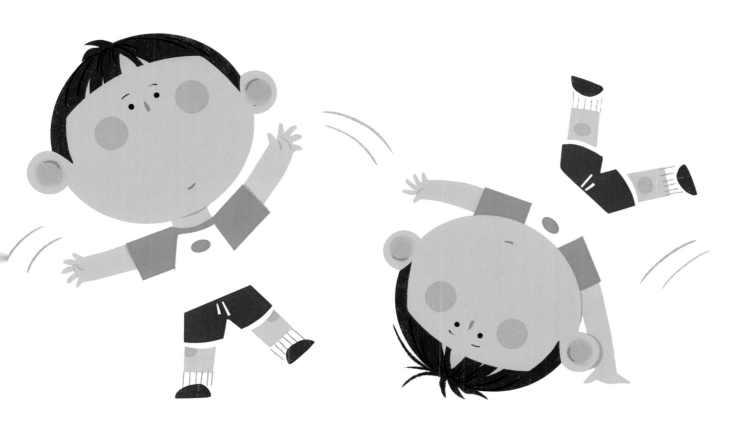

D
is for Duck Walk
squat and walk, quack quack

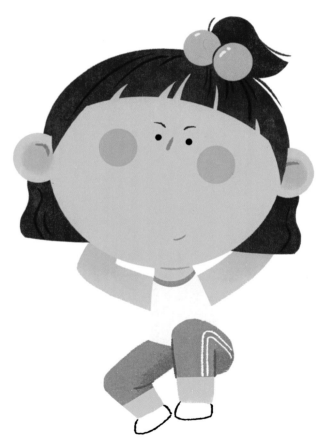

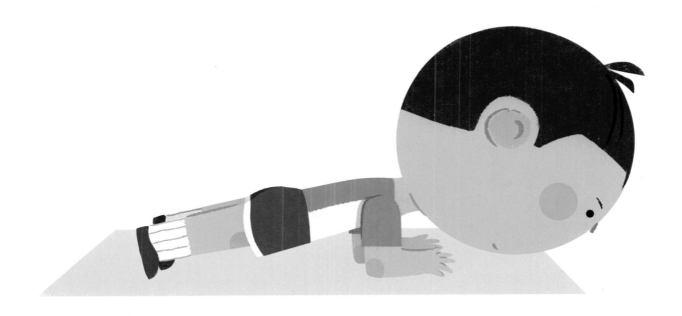

E is for Elbow Plank

elbows on the floor and balance on your tiptoes

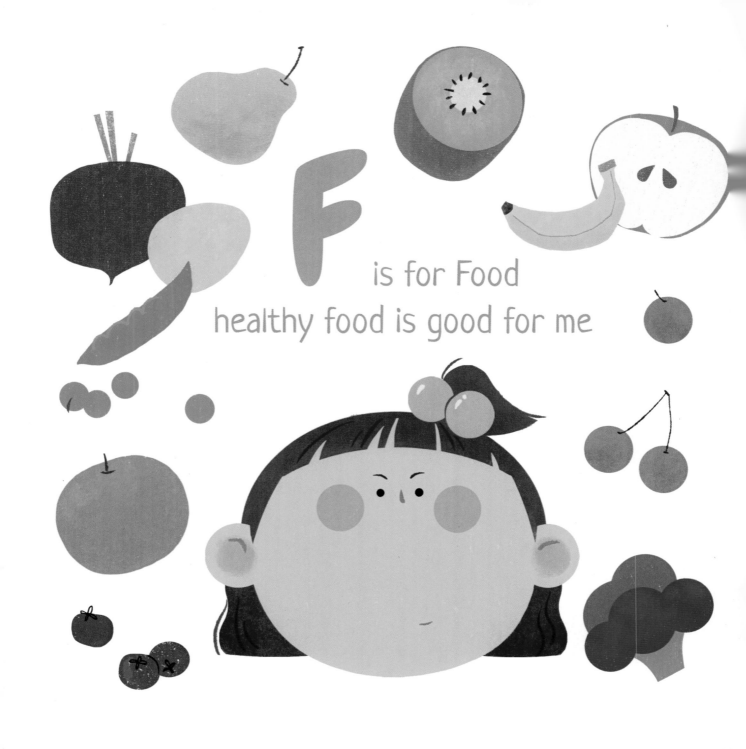

F is for Food
healthy food is good for me

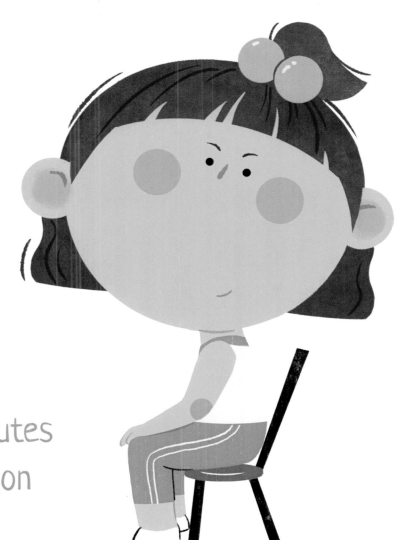

G is for Glutes
the muscle I sit on

H is for Handstand
standing on my hands

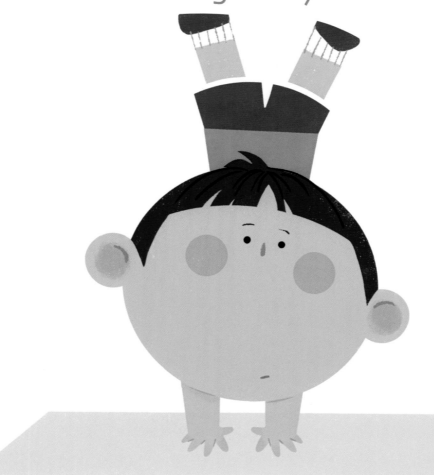

I

is for Inchworm
touch your toes and move like a caterpillar

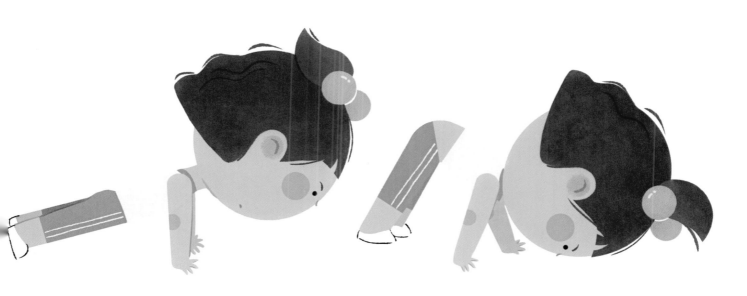

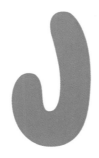 is for Jumping Jacks

"pencil"   "teepee"   "pencil"

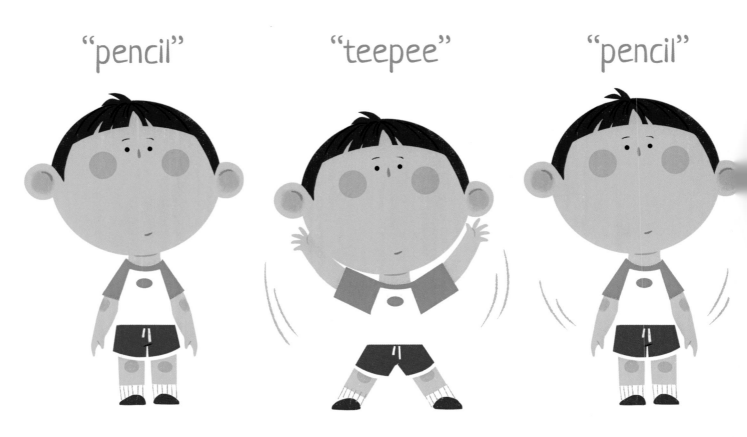

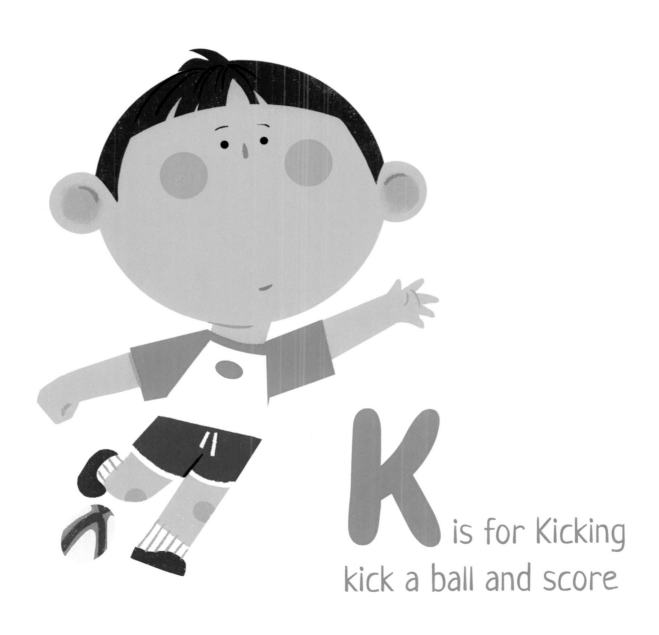

K is for Kicking
kick a ball and score

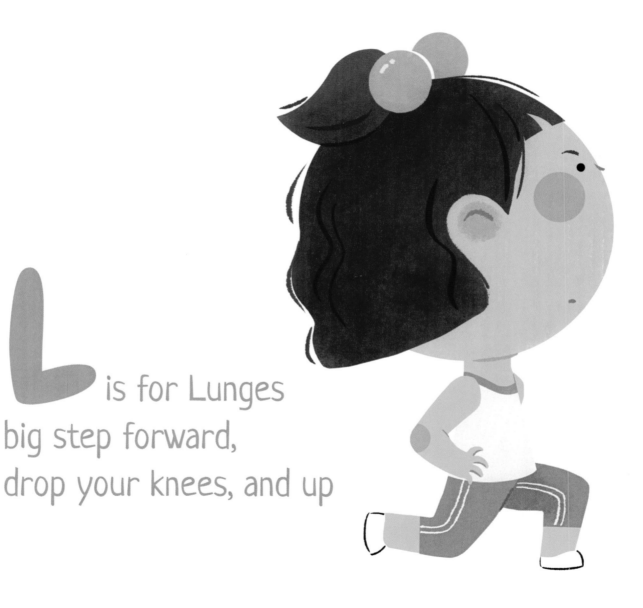

L is for Lunges
big step forward,
drop your knees, and up

M is for Mountain Climber
one foot forward and back,
one foot forward and back

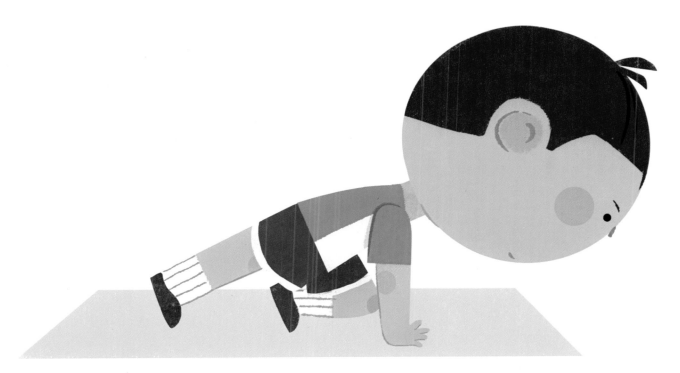

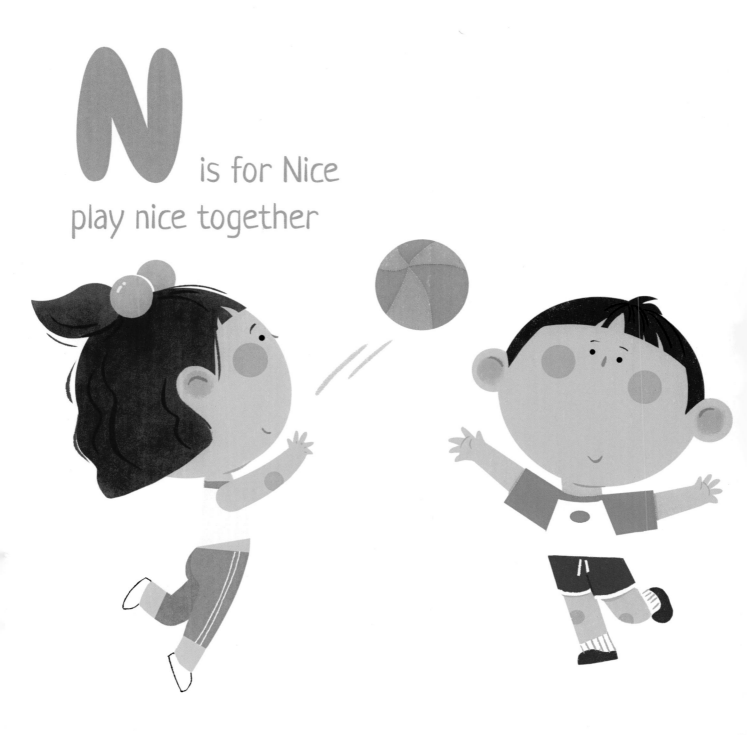

N is for Nice
play nice together

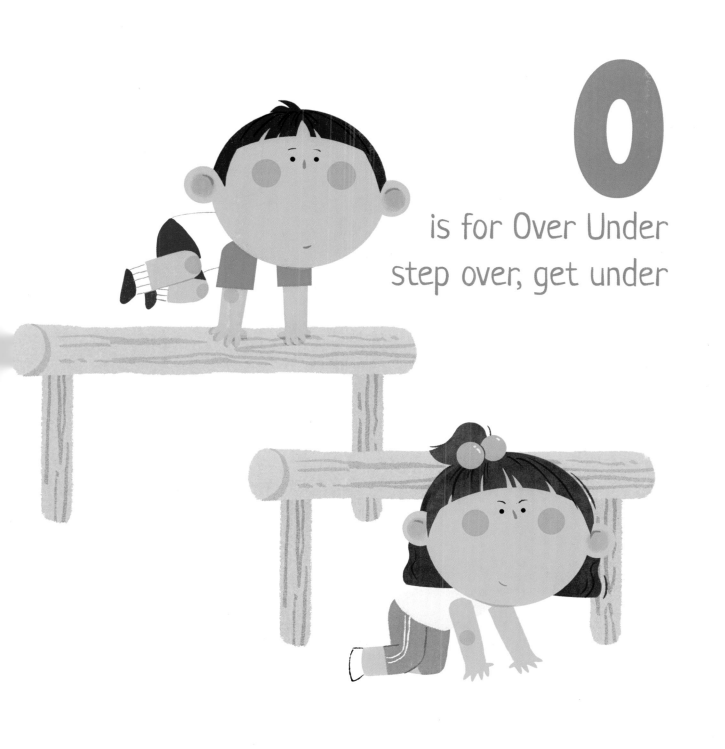

O is for Over Under
step over, get under

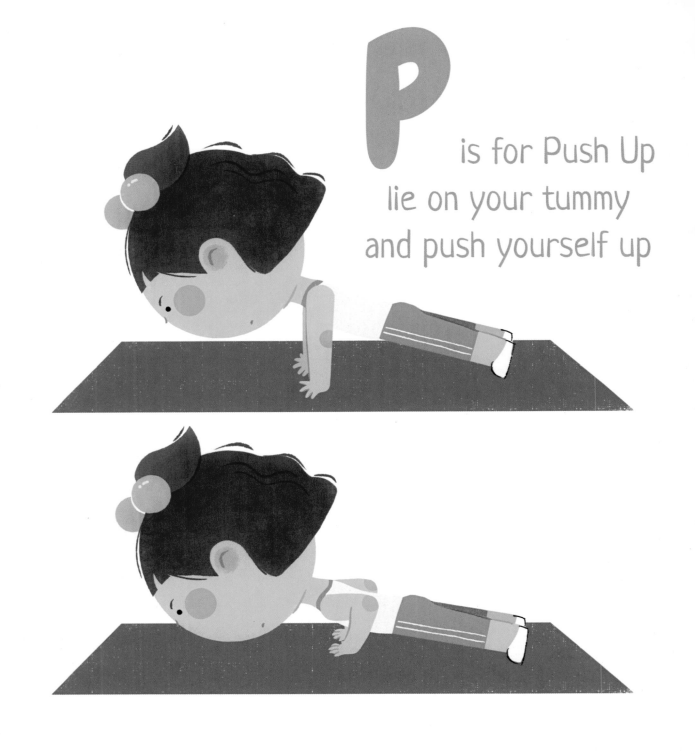

P is for Push Up
lie on your tummy
and push yourself up

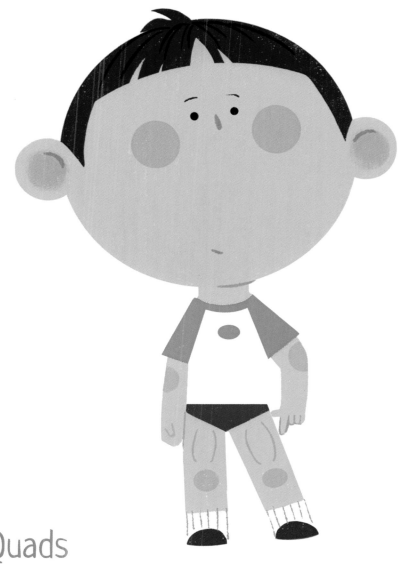

Q is for Quads
the muscle on the front of my thigh

R

is for Running
as fast as you can

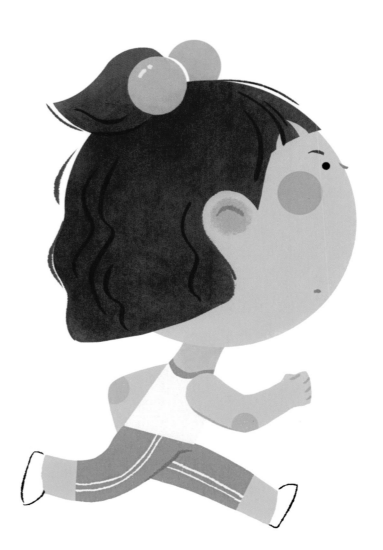

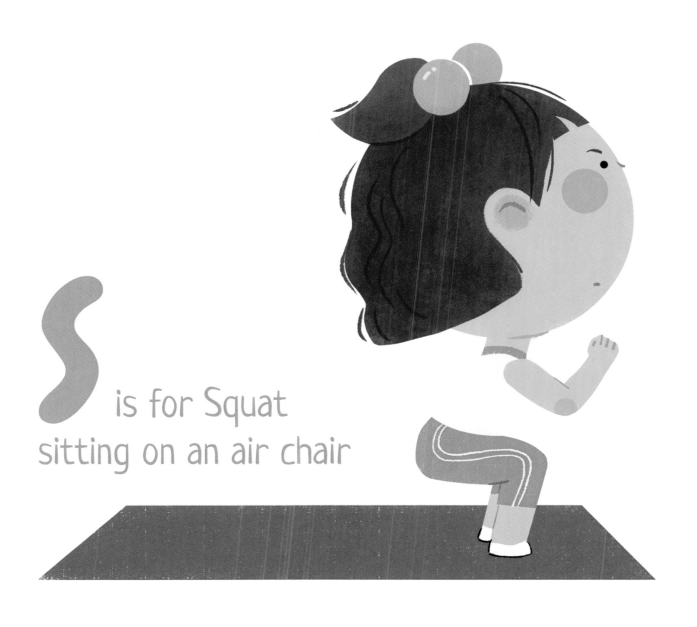

is for Squat
sitting on an air chair

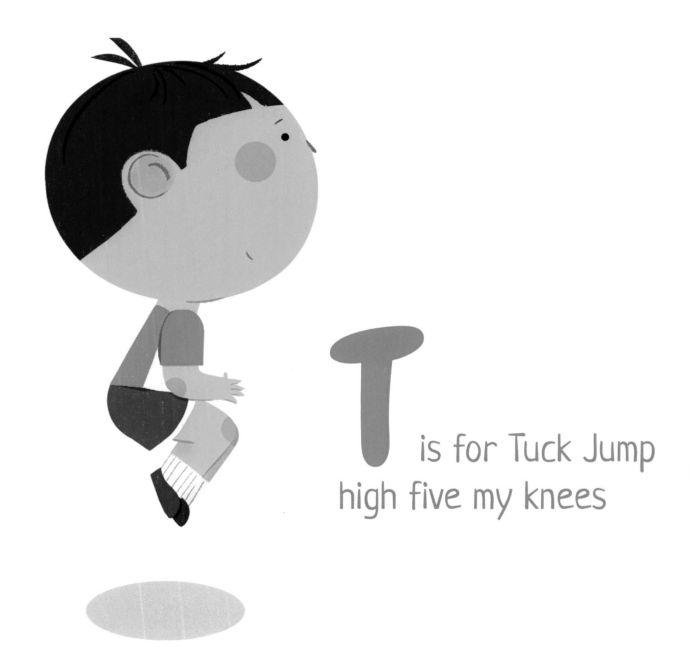

T is for Tuck Jump
high five my knees

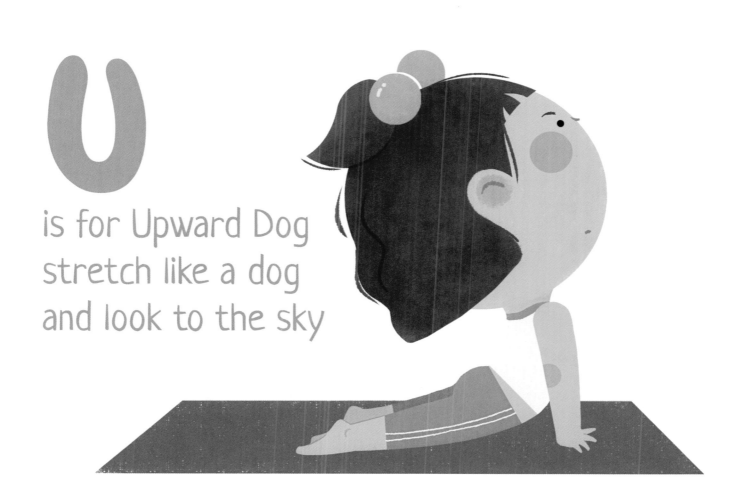

is for Upward Dog
stretch like a dog
and look to the sky

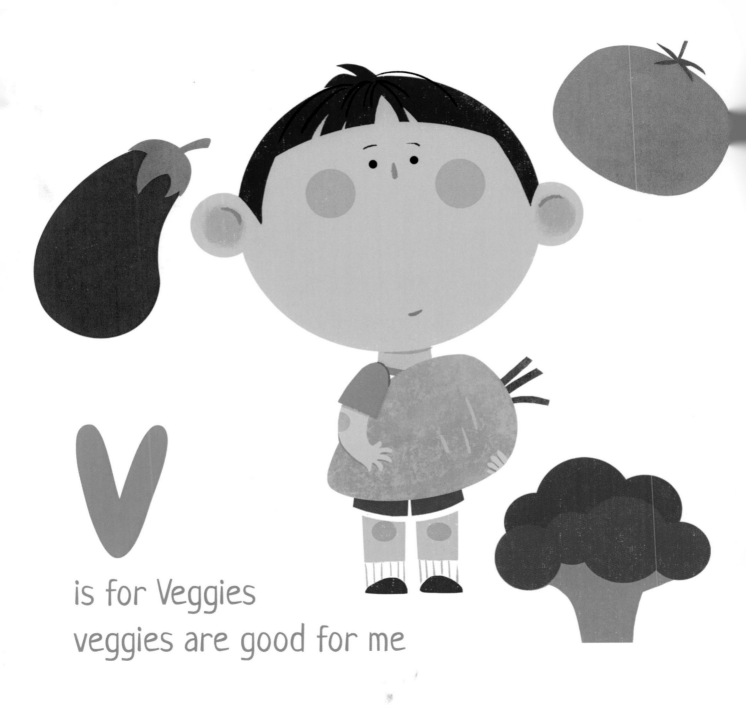

V is for Veggies
veggies are good for me

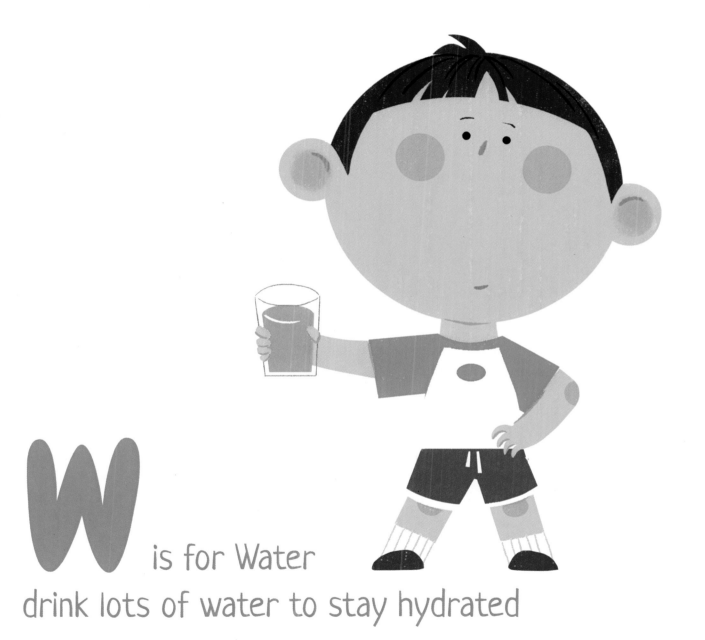

W is for Water
drink lots of water to stay hydrated

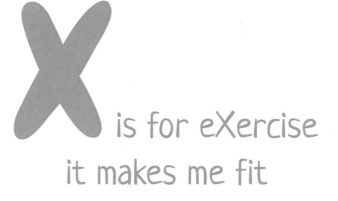

X is for eXercise
it makes me fit

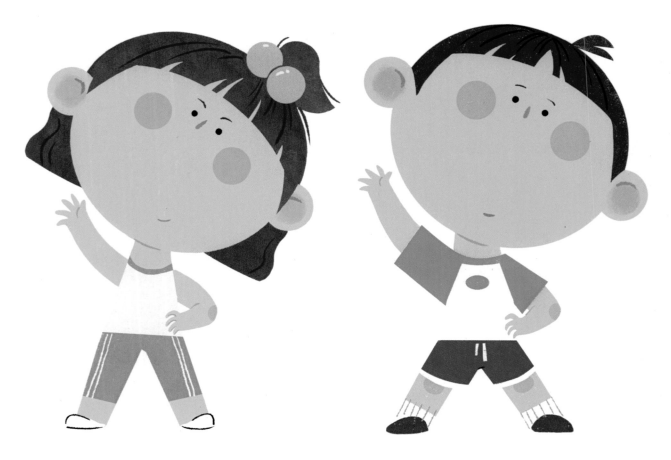

Y is for Yoga
breath in and out and stretch

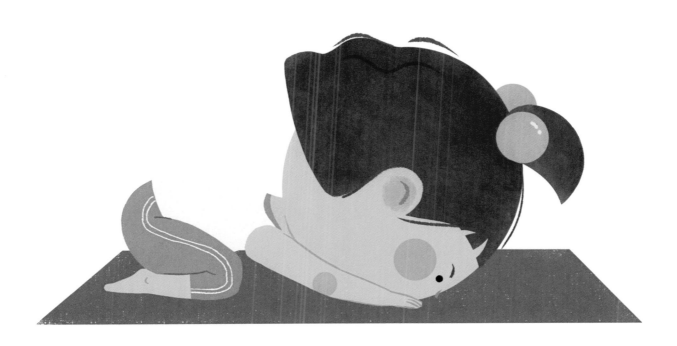

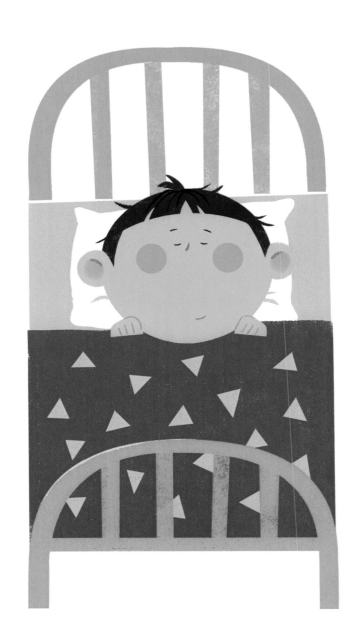

z

is for zzz sleep
the rest that I need

Made in the USA
Monee, IL
23 February 2023

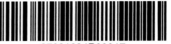

27621684R00017